WEIGHT LOSS
THE EASY WAY

12 STEPS TO SUCCESS

A Weight-Loss Program That Brings Results!

Mac Isaya

ISBN: 143825086X
ISBN-13: 9781438250861

CONTENTS

Disclaimer: No part of this book is meant to be a substitute for professional medical advice. This book is for educational purposes only.

If you need to check or change your Basal Metabolic Rate or cholesterol, or you have another health issue, consult a health practitioner first.

Before taking food supplements, consult health practitioner regarding potential allergies.

INTRODUCTION

This book describes EZWAY12, a realistic program for weight loss! It is the direct result of fifteen years of personal search and experience, based on my frustration when regular weight loss programs did not work.

I recently read about five "miracle" foods that guarantee weight loss: apples, tomatoes, salmon, eggs, and something else like some nuts. Can you imagine waking up and saying, "Honey, make me a boiled egg with tomato." C'mon!

The articles about weight loss that come out every three month or so show the desperation and frustration with regular diet programs. If the well-known programs worked, otherwise obesity would not be the problem in America that it is.

If a weight loss schedule does not fit your current lifestyle, you will not do it, just like I would not. This program is based on a *realistic* regimen of exercises and minimum imposition on your body. It is easy and enjoyable.

Say that you want to learn karate, so you go to a karate school. You would want the sensei to be a black belt with many years of experience. However, imagine that you come to the training and see people like you—lawyers , doctors, carpenters, firefighters—all teaching each other karate. That would be nonsense!

That is exactly what happens with weight loss in the United States. Because there are so many people who can't manage their weight, you find great public interest, interest from the medical community, and interest from people who otherwise would not express interest at all, as they are all trying to show that they know something about weight loss. They assume a perfect world scenario, where everybody can and will do what they are asked to do: eat less and exercise more.

That is not the case in the real world. EZWAY12 gives you real-world scenarios with a real-life action plan.

After so many years of research about weight loss, why is it that the experts cannot say what works? It is because they are not personally involved; they are conditioned by orthodox medical school – they don't look 'outside the box'.

The only miracle they hope is that a medical technology will be developed that allows us to silence the genes responsible for weight gain. Someday? When?

Experts write lengthy books about weight loss, but they miss the most important point. People are not Olympians!

I could write a five-hundred-page book on this subject, because I have more than enough information and knowledge to do so, but is that what you want? You want meaningful information that leads you to action. I have many books on weight loss that I ordered and did not read past first chapter— because it's the same old story of weight loss the hard way.

Ninety five percent of people do that, and 45 percent of people who buy a book don't even open it.

This information was extracted from experience and is presented to you in a form that is easy to use.

I wanted to make this program different. I want you to read it and to use it 100 percent , and I want you to enjoy what you are doing 100 percent , because that is the only way that you will stick with it!

CHAPTER 1

How many times have you tried—and failed—to lose weight? I have tried it all. I've been on diets, and it seemed like lost weight but I had not, or I lost weight and gained it back.

I exercised, and my legs and joints hurt. Jogging when you are overweight, as many therapists will tell you, is dangerous, because it puts pressure on your joints.

How many hard-earned dollars have you spent on weight-loss programs? Would you pay $149.00 for a book, delivered right to your mailbox, that contains *real* advice gathered from fifteen years of study? I thought that the suggested price was ridiculously high.

But a lot of people pay $149.00 for visit to a doctor!

"$14.90" and not a cent more for my service.I have been in your situation. I tried all the diet programs, and none of them worked.The programs that you see advertised on TV don't work. If they did, you could see a different culture, because *everybody* would use the program and lose weight.

The medical community in America does not know what to do about obesity, which has become the greatest problem in the country, second only to drug abuse. Most medical practitioners suggest primitive life changes like jogging and eating less. They did not work for me, and they will not work for you.

I used to be overweight , and now I'm within a normal weight range, but it took fifteen years of trial and error.

That experience that led me to discover the system that works: EZWAY12.

It consists of twelve distinct principles that help you lose weight even when you are asleep. It is easy on your body.

Most books about weight loss go on and on, give many unimportant details, and brag about the promised results. They give hundreds of testimonies to convince you of the writer's opinion.

These are what I call "convincer metaprogram" books. They give you a thousand reasons to be convinced of one important thing. They do not simply give that advice up front, because the 170-page book would be four pages. Think of corporate reports or confidential memos that contain no pictures, no testimonies, only facts. That is what you will find in this book.

I don't want to convince you or anybody. You are the only one who can convince yourself.

If you need testimonies of presidents, you will not find them here. No testimonies, no fancy images just principles for action.

I tell you what works, based on my fifteen years of trial and error.

I give you facts and explanations. Most books on weight loss are overloaded with useless information, and you may never read beyond the first chapter. This book you can actually *use*.

PRINCIPLE #1: YOU WILL LOSE WEIGHT ONLY IF IT IS EASY ON YOUR BODY AND PSYCHE.

I've learned from experience that people abandon any program that requires "working" on it.

Anything that requires hard labor makes your body and mind rebel. Your psyche, or psychological disposition, has a certain degree of compliance with the way you live and your circumstances.

Let's say that you like to hang out with your friends. You love the activity, and that's why you do it. You go to Burger King, Jack-in-the-Box, or Starbucks, and you enjoy eating out there. It's part of your life. You drink coffee and eat donuts at work with your colleagues.

You don't do these activities by yourself, and because they are enjoyable, releasedopamine in your brain. Dopamine is a neurohormone released in certain parts of brain in response to or in expectation of reward. Anything that gets in the way of that activity will be avoided.

Until scientists discover something that mimics dopamine, people will continue to gain weight.

Do what you do, eat what you want, and enjoy it, knowing that you can achieve your goal of losing weight.

CHAPTER 2

You already have the first and most important principle of the EZWAY12 program. Do only the activities that you enjoy doing, because that's your only insurance that this program will last. The philosophy of "no pain, no gain" is only for Olympic athletes and doesn't work in real life.

You might say, "Okay, I must get used to this unconventional idea that I can and will lose weight without hard work." It's strange, but it's true.

As I said, the medical community can't agree on what causes obesity and how to deal with it. The situation in some states is so severe that members of Congress asked the Food and Drug Administration to give priority status to technologies and drugs aimed at combating the obesity problem (which itself is the cause of other major health problems).

Even the most expensive diet programs give the same advice as your doctor:
Eat less, diet,
exercise more,
establish goals,
check on the outcome,
monitor your progress, and do
aerobic conditioning.
The list goes on.

Some have more exotic explanations: You are genetically predisposed, you gain weight after you stop smoking, you eat when you are happy, you eat when you are depressed, or you gain weight because you go out with friends and binge.

What are you supposed to do? Give up all your friends?

No way. You can have your pie and eat it too.

Do what you like, eat what you want, and you will still lose weight with EZWAY12.

PRINCIPLE #2: DO REVERSE JUMPING.

This is not an exercise that you do with an instructor at the gym. It's an exercise that I developed, and it is so easy that I do it one thousand to one hundred thousand times a day. You can start with one hundred. Anytime you have about thirty seconds free, you can *want* to do this exercise even though you are not obligated to.

What is reverse jumping, and why is it so important?

You know what jumping is. You jump upward, but reverse jumping does the opposite. Stand up and "jump downward." You jump while standing on your feet; your feet do not leave the ground.

You can start by doing three to four reverse jumps per second and increase to five to ten jumps per second (or you can stick with the slow rate).

At first reverse jumping may feel odd, but once you get used to it, you can enjoy the process. It's easy and fun.

Try this: Imagine that you have one-thousand-pound boots on your feet, and you need to jump, not just walk. Bend your knees a little, and jump without letting your feet leave the ground.

I do up to one hundred thousand reverse jumps a day, and it's so easy and enjoyable that I don't even keep count.

If you do the reverse jump exercise fast enough, you will have to do what I call fractured breathing. It is also very candid lung exercise.

While you jump, you inhale on counts one through five. These counts would be air by fractures. Count to five and exhale in fractures. Fracture is a medical term that usually describes something broken or parted, such as "fractured bone". Picture your breath as a whole and divide it into parts. It's that simple.

Why is this exercise so important? The body functions with the help of the internal organs, and the kidneys play a crucial role. Aside from cleansing water and extracting urine, they regulate the alkaline balance of blood plasma. Aldosterone regulates emissions of erythropoietin, which regulate how many erythrocytes you have, and renine regulates systemic blood pressure. Erythrocytes, or red blood cells, are vital because they carry oxygen to all body tissues.However, there is a slight problem.

You cannot exercise your internal organs. Your muscles and bones get exercise, as does your heart when it acts as a pump, but not so for your kidneys, liver, brain, and other organs.

Many doctors have given testimonials on the positive effects of jumping and trampolining. I took this type of exercise a step further, making it faster, easier, more enjoyable, and more relaxed, because you don't leave the ground.

When I started doing this exercise and included it in my regimen, I didn't realize the benefits of healthier kidneys. Since then, I regularly measured my erythrocytes and erythropoietin levels, and they were always up. That meant more oxygen for every cell of my body.

Even though I was still overweight, I started to feel much better and more energized. That alone gave me the strength and desire to do things and go places, to explore what I am capable of further, and even to write a book about weight loss.

Other positive "side" effects include: better teeth, hair, nail, and skin appearance. Do the reverse jumping exercise in the way that it's convenient, and you are doing it right.

CHAPTER 3

You have probably noticed already how easy it is to follow this program. Unlike other diet programs that ask you to do hard work, such as exercising in a gym, this program is easy, understandable, and enjoyable.

You have probably also realized that this is an exclusive book. The principles found here won't be found anywhere else.

I started like everybody else. I started jogging to lose weight. I stopped meeting with friends, which made me angry and upset, and as a result, I ate even more. I went swimming and hiking, and I lifted weights. My knees and back started to hurt, and I was not losing weight.

I went on different diets such as a highprotein diet, a low-carb diet, to mention a few. My metabolism dropped, and I ate less but still gained weight. My doctor suggested that I eat less and exercise more (but only after knee surgery).

I thought, "There's got to be a better way."

I started studying the literature to discover principles that made sense and got results, principles that would work, and principles that I could easily accommodate into my life and would enjoy.

That's how I realized that, like many others, you will not stick to a program that produces no results and leads to frustration. You stick to a program that is easy to implement *and* that produces results at the same time.

That is why I want to give you the principles of my weight-loss program, EZWAY12.

Numerous studies have been done on the effect of aerobics, and the number of studies on the positive effect of anaerobics is about the same. Some doctors believe in jogging, and others believe in interval training. If you do either one long enough, you will be injured. I know that for a fact.

Years ago, I heard of a study on walking, and I discovered a type of walking that gave far superior results than "simple" walking. "Finnish walking" (named for Finland) is done by walking with ski poles, or with sticks that are up to waistline in length.

The data stunned me. The effect of Finnish walking showed double the efficacy of regular exercise, such as jogging. I thought there must be something more. Doctors tried to explain that the results were from longer steps and arm movement, but I was not convinced. Something didn't add up. I researched the calories burned by skiing at the same pace. In this sport, people had much wider steps and the added hand movement, but the results were low and didn't add up to Finnish walking.

I dug further and learned the one element that contributes to burning many more calories, almost as many as averaged interval training. I call it the "Swirl Exercise."

PRINCIPLE #3: SWIRL EXERCISE.

If you stand up you can turn your torso approximately at ninety degree angle to the right and the same to the left – hat would count a full swirl.

When you do Finnish walking with sticks, you have to swirl your torso. You don't do this while "simple" walking, and you don't do it while skiing. What else could differentiate those exercises? Nothing.

Years later, I found a product in a sporting equipment store that worked on this principle. It was a metallic disc that you stood on, and you swirled your torso around a vertical axis periodically.

I don't know the name of the product, but "simple" walking around your house while swirling the torso burns calories.

CHAPTER 4

Your doctor is your best friend, and parasites are your worst enemies.

If you are like me, you are skeptical of doctors. How could someone charge so much for treatment or visit? Our healthcare system is bloated out of proportion and there is nothing you and I can do about it. However, there are good health professionals that will help you. I assume that you have regular checkups and visit your doctor whenever you are in pain. Do yourself a favor, and the next time that you see your doctor, ask to see a parasitologist: a doctor who deals with parasites.

Most people don't know when they have parasites, which can be as simple as candida or as complex as lower bowel worms.

Among other things, they cause overtoxicity, which changes your alkaline-acidic balance. As the result of that, your Basal Metabolic Rate (BMR) lowers to deal with fat-soluble and water-soluble waste, and your body uses stored fat as a protection mechanism against over-acidity.

PRINCIPLE #4: GET RID OF PARASITES.

During your next visit to a clinic, see a parasitologist. He or she will explain to you why this important problem overlooked.

If you find that you have a parasite, work with your doctor to treat it, and schedule a follow-up checkup.

On the EZWAY12 program, nothing should stand in your way to achieving your desired results, not even organisms that may have lived with you for years. The micro-organisms and worms like to eat, and their primary source of energy is glucose. That's why no matter how much you eat, they take their part and leave the rest for your body to absorb.

A few years back, a bookcalled *Miracle pH* was published. Many of the ideas behind the book's thesis was that overacidity within the body causes huge problems. Though I believe that this problem is overstated, the underlying idea is that your body acidity needs to be within a normal range.

Parasites mostly live in acidic environments, and they tend to produce acidic waste, making the situation worse.

Acidity makes your body store fat and is not good for your bones and teeth; the calcium, which is primarily alkaline, gets depleted to neutralize it. It can even cause serious medical conditions down the road, such as osteoporosis – porous bones with decreased mineral density which increases risks of bone fractures and arthritis – joint failure.

Testing and treating parasites is easy. Do yourself and your body a favor and get rid of parasites. Nothing should stand in your way to your goals, and parasites are one of two issues that prevent weight loss with EZWAY12.

CHAPTER 5

I was stunned when I recently saw a program on a mainstream TV channel about obesity in America.

It included color-coded graphics to show how different states had changed from white (where less that 5 percent of population was obese) to red (where more than 30 percent of the population was obese).

The worst situation is in Missouri, but the fact is that in every state, 25 to 30 percent of the population is obese.

The concern is growing, but we are on the wrong path. Don't blame fast food or your way of life; your way of life, if you are like most of us, is perfectly normal. You want to enjoy life, and food is one of your greatest pleasures.

Let's talk about your lymph system, which is the body's drainage system. It is composed of a network of vessels and small structures called lymph nodes. The lymph vessels convey excess fluid, collected from all over the body, back into the blood. Along the way, these fluids percolate through the lymph nodes so that they can be filtered. Harmful organisms are trapped and destroyed by specialized white blood cells, called *lymphocytes,* that are present in these nodes. Lymphocytes are added to the lymph that flows out of nodes and back to the bloodstream.

The lymph system is important because it manufactures *antibodies.* Antibodies are specialized proteins that the body produces in response to invasion by a foreign substance. The process of antibody formation begins when an antigen, which is a molecule that triggers the production of special antibodies, stimulates specialized lymphocytes, called B cells, into action.

Antibodies counteract by combining with the antigen to render it harmless.

You heart pumps your blood, but the lymph system has no pump! The only way it moves is by exercise.

You have to get rid of anything that keeps unnecessary waste in your body, and if the "sewage system" is not functioning well or is overloaded, the system gets clogged.

Walking and running can provide the pumping, but what if I told you that there is an easier, more efficient way to regularly clean your lymph system?

That's what this EZWAY12 program is about: making life easier for you, not harder.

PRINCIPLE #5: "IRON" YOUR BODY WHEN YOU WAKE UP.

What is the period of the day that you move the least? It's when you are sleeping. By morning, your lymph system has accumulated some portion of waste—it has worked hard to keep your system pure and your body safe.

Your lymph system, or at least most of it, is right under your skin. The first thing I do after I wake up is caress the skin of my body with my palms. I call this the "Ironing exercise."

Imagine that your palm is an ultra–modern iron that comforts your skin, and you need to iron all of your skin—palms,chest,legs, back, everywhere possible.

When you "iron" your body, you get your body's lymph moving, and this helps your lymph system to get rid of waste.

Do this exercise when you wake up or whenever you feel like doing it, and combine it with other exercises from your EZWAY12 program whenever possible. It only takes a minute or two to do each one of them.

CHAPTER 6

You probably noticed that unlike any other program, EZWAY12 doesn't ask you to exercise, diet, monitor your calories, monitor your weight, or restrict anything in life.

That's why the EZWAY12 program works. It is efficient and readily available, and the actions are easy.

Ten to fifteen years ago, it was rare for Eskimos (native people living in Alaska) to suffer from obesity or associated problems. One reason, as studies show, was that they live in a nature-friendly environment, but over time, they lost the motivation to live like their parents and grandparents, and they got sucked into the challenges of obesity.

PRINCIPLE #6: TAKE COLD SHOWERS.

Numerous studies show that exposure to cold (air or water) increases your BMR.

When I started to incorporate this principle in my life, I simply lowered the temperature of the water when I showered. It's that simple! If you cannot tolerate cold water right away, make the water a bit cooler with each shower. Continued progress is more important than immediate action.

Cold water is much more stimulating than warm water for blood circulation, and it increases the rate of your body's immune response.

CHAPTER 7

You now know how harmful microorganisms and parasites can be and the effects they have in building waste, excess fluid, and fat in your body.

Another process causes excess fluid to accumulate and makes your body maintain that fluid regardless of your desire to lose it.

You can run or swim until you're blue in the face, but your body will maintain the fluids and fat that are necessary to protect you.

There has been much talk about the effect of the nuclear disaster in Fukushima. For Japan, the radiation exposure is enormous and harmful, but it's also true for the West Coast of the United States.

The largest threat is the exposure to harmful doses of iodine, which affects the thyroid gland. Even more harmful can be exposure to particles of uranium, cesium, strontium, plutonium, and an even more dangerous substance referred to as dioxin. A single molecule of dioxin can produce more damage, continuously, than the effects of air, water, and land metal exposure combined. The World Health Organization, which governs health policies around the world, has put dioxin on its list of "Ten most harmful pollutants."

Once these large, metallic particles and pollutants are in your body, they can't get out by themselves, and the amount of oxidative damage can be enormous.

In the modern world, the risk of exposure to toxins and heavier particles is growing.

After the Fukushima blast, a two- year of supply of iodine replacement was wiped out of the market in matter of days (the selling price on soared from $3 to $250). Acquiring iodine is the easiest part; minimizing toxic exposure is hard.

PRINCIPLE #7: START A FIBER CLEANSING PROGRAM TO REMOVE HEAVIER PARTICLES THAT DISTURB AND IRRITATE YOUR CELLS.

The next step in this easy weightloss program is minimizing toxic exposure and getting waste out of your body with the help of *adsorptionists* and *absorptionists*.

The most well-known absorptionist is activated carbon, but from my experience, it is not as satisfactory because one needs to saturate your digestive track with it for the carbon to work.

A better substance is called *lignum vitae*. It is an adsorptionist—it binds to the heavier molecules. Being a complex fiber, it carries the heavy molecule iron (strontium) out of the body.

For me, *lignum vitae* was the most complicated part of cleansing and the one that produced the best results. If you can't find a *lignum vitae* tablet producer, write to me. Be sure to consult your physician about allergy testing.

I don't want to add to the vitamin-mineral-hormone frenzy, but I tried it all: high doses of vitamins, low doses of minerals, DHEAs (testosterone precursor hormone), resveratrol (nutrient extracted from grape seeds), etc. I am skeptical of intrusive therapies unless they are justified. Fiber cleansing is not an intrusive therapy, because almost all of fiber you intake is eliminated though the bowel, which then starts to function much better.

My conclusion is that nothing works better than fiber adsorption.

Get *lignum vitae* or, with the help of your nutritionist, find some other fiber-adsorption component to safely cleanse your system of heavier metal particles and enjoy the result.

CHAPTER 8

This program is popular and enjoyable because it is so easy. If it is easy, you will stick to it, and if it is not easy, you will find an excuse to abandon it.

Next I want to describe what I call "Tensing."

PRINCIPLE #8: USE THE POWER OF TENSING.

Have you ever seen how an animal (such as your cat) exercises?

It performs what can be called "a cat's stretch."

Stand up with your hands stretched up as much as you can. You don't even have to stand up to do this exercise—you can do it in bed!

Or imagine yourself on a surfboard catching the wave. Even if you never surfed, you have seen surfers and may noticed how tensed they are on the board. The exercise of standing on a surfboard is a good one. Tensing is important to keep your spinal cord in good condition, and your spinal cord is the most integral part of your central nervous system.

Bring your hands up with your toes on the floor, and hold the position tight for five to ten seconds. That's it.

You can do this exercise anywhere, much like the surfer's. Focus on the spinal cord as if a force has compressed it. Watch how dogs and cats exercise; they tend to stretch by tensing.

Tensing is also great for your BMR, because it helps to work your internal muscles.

CHAPTER 9

Remember how I said that there is nothing that you cannot eat? I mean that! If you like the food at Burger King, go for it, especially if you enjoy it with your friends.

One food deserves special attention, and I'm talking about beer.

I used to drink beer all the time. It relaxes you, your friends drink it, and you enjoy it. When I encountered the facts about beer, the facts were plain and simple. The yeast in beer will not let you lose weight.

PRINCIPLE #9: AVOID BEER.

Beer has the highest concentration of yeast. It lets the candida, which is harmful bacteria grow, so you are growing a "candida plantation," and candida creates acidity.

If you are interested in what candida does to overall well-being, read the book *Miracle pH*. It explains this issue scientifically.

How are you going to enjoy a game or evening with your friends if everybody else is drinking beer and you are not?

Make a smarter move. If social drinking is inevitable, drink a glass of red wine. Instead of sipping bottle after bottle of beer, I now ask for a glass of California red wine.

Notice that I don't ask you to cut drinking alcohol to zero or to eliminate it from your diet. If you feel restricted as to what you can or cannot eat, change will not work out in the long term. The only program that will work long term for you is the one that fits easily with your lifestyle.

The one beverage that you don't need is beer.

Upgrade your taste to higher level of sophistication, and ask for a glass of wine instead.

CHAPTER 10

Another important subject relative to this program is ballet.

Have you ever seen a ballet dancer who is overweight? I haven't. What do they do? Do they jog many miles?

If you watch ballet, you find a couple of interesting things.

First, ballet dancers do a lot of tensing when performing. They also do a lot of swirls; they turn their torso back and forth while the rest of their body is still.

They also do an important exercise that helps you to lose weight efficiently, which I call "Balancing."

PRINCIPLE #10: ENJOY THE POWER OF BALANCING WITH THE "GRIZZLY BEAR" EXERCISE.

Balancing is great for working your internal muscles. Your body will work the muscles that keep you from falling.

Most people cannot perform balancing in the same way as a professional ballet dancer, and they don't need to.

I made it easy. Stand on one leg and then on the other: left, right.

Imagine a grizzly bear moving around in the woods.

How would a grizzly bear balance on its back legs? Do the same.

As you get used to this exercise, your steps can become slower and wider, and you can improvise, balancing forward and backward and using your arms together.

Balancing allows you to burn fat, and it is easy and enjoyable!

CHAPTER 11

One factor that plays an important role in your overall anxiety level is the amount of time you sleep.

You should sleep no less than eight hours each night (eight to ten hours on the weekend).

You may know that hormones like melatonin are produced only at night. Equally important is the fact that if you cannot completely relax and restore your body from your activity during the daytime, fatigue will build up over time, causing you more stress and anxiety.

PRINCIPLE #11: GET EIGHT HOURS OF SLEEP EACH NIGHT.

Relaxation does not have to be done only at night. Find a relaxation practice that suits you. Good ones include tai chi, meditation, yoga, and listening to relaxing music.

Being well rested and relaxed will add to benefits of the EZWAY12 program and the principles you now know.

CHAPTER 12

You are making great progress here! You are on the last chapter of EZWAY12 program and on track to successful weight loss.

By now, you know that being overweight is not about fructose, dieting, hamburgers, jogging, exercise, or your Body-Mass Index. It's not about "more fruit, less salt," and so on.

Don't believe someone who says that being overweight is inevitable or that it is genetic. If I can lose weight, so can you!

By reading this book, you are becoming psychologically fit, you know which habits to adopt, how to eliminate the obstacles that keep you from having your desired body, and how to do easy, enjoyable exercises.

You are on the right path! It's like having a secret weapon that you got for very little money.

What else remains in the EZWAY12 program?

Relationships.

I do not mean only sex (although sex burns more calories than most exercise), but being in a relationship will help you to improve from the inside, to keep your promises, and to hold yourself to a higher standard.

This is an area where many people experience frustration, just as they do with weight loss.

There are couples who are overweight and still love each other, and that is great. There are also many people who are frustrated and alone and do not know what to do.

That was the case for me. I read many books on how to attract a loved one.

I read books on "Mars and Venus," being an "alpha male," the secret signs that women send to men, ""it's all for the money" theory," and science of neuro –linguistic programming

These theories try to develop Freudian theory and miss the major point: how would I maintain the relationship with someone who I love and who loves me?

For example, say that you know the signs of attraction in a woman or man or you send (or receive) those signals. How do you know that you will not lose the attraction ten minutes later?

According to the alphamale theory, you just become a weightlifter in a cool shirt and that would do it. You and I both know that it is not the case.

It's not also about the money, because money can't buy love. I can buy intimacy but definitely not love.

Through personal experience, I found that there is only one thing to remember about starting or building a relationship.

It is easy to tear down a relationship and hard to build one, but once you know this principle, building a relationship will be easy for you.

PRINCIPLE #12: BUILD THE RELATIONSHIP; BUILD THE STORY.

Let's say that at "time X," you don't have a relationship. You want to go from there to "time Y" when you have a healthy, sustainable relationship.

You have to start and build your relationship around events that are part of your shared story, the story that the other person can relate to even when you are not around.

Human beings relate to each other or to something in the future only if we have experienced such events in the past or if we imagine that we *will* experience those events (based on a promise). Of those factors, the former is much stronger.

If you are a man, you don't have to wear a three-piece suit or stand on your wallet to attract someone or maintain a relationship with another person. You won't need to recognize if a man or woman is ready to connect with you.

The easiest way to connect is through building rapport based on commonalities.

For example, if you are walking in the park with your dog, talk with other people about dogs. If you are in the bar, talk about drinks. You get the idea—find something that connects you.

This strategy works only at the start of the relationship while becoming acquainted. You can't meet the person again and talk about the same things and expect results. You need to "build a story" of shared events.

Did you pick up that weird-looking flower along sidewalk? Did you forget the coffee cup on the roof of your car when you came out of a fancy café?

"Crazy" events like these allow you to relate back in time and extrapolate how your relationship will develop in the future.

SUMMARY

Now you have the twelve principles that will put you on the road to successful weight loss!

Principle #1: Only do exercises that are easy and enjoyable.

Principle #2: Do reverse jumping.

Principle #3: Do the swirl exercise.

Principle #4: Get rid of parasites.

Principle #5: "Iron" your body to propel your lymph system.

Principle #6: Take cold showers.

Principle #7: Start a fiber cleansing program.

Principle #8: Use the power of tensing.

Principle #9: Avoid beer. Principle #10: Enjoy the power of balancing with the "grizzly bear" exercise.

Principle #11: Get eight hours of sleep each night.

Principle #12: Build a relationship.

This is not the end of your weight-loss adventure but the beginning of improving from the inside. I wish you the best on your road to success!

www.ingramcontent.com/pod-product-compliance
Lightning Source LLC
Chambersburg PA
CBHW052023280526
45793CB00005B/1098